THE PATH TO A HAPPIER LIFE:

Making Simple Changes for Healthy Habits

Alberto L. Wilson

Welcome to "The Path to a Happier Life: Making Simple Changes for Healthy Habits." In our fast-paced and demanding world, it's easy to get caught up in the whirlwind of responsibilities and neglect our well-being. However, true happiness stems from nurturing our physical, mental, and emotional health. This book is designed to guide you on a transformative journey toward a happier and more fulfilling life through the power of simple changes and healthy habits.

Once upon a time, in a bustling city filled with people chasing after their dreams, there lived a young woman named Sarah. Sarah seemed to have it all – a successful career, a beautiful apartment, and a wide circle of friends. However, despite her external accomplishments, she couldn't shake off a lingering sense of discontentment. There was a void within her, an emptiness that whispered, "There must be more to life than this."

One evening, as Sarah sat in her favorite coffee shop, contemplating the meaning of true happiness, she noticed an elderly couple sitting across from her. They held hands, their eyes twinkling with affection and warmth. Their laughter filled the air, and it was as if their souls were dancing in harmony. Sarah couldn't help but be captivated by their joy.

Intrigued by their evident happiness, Sarah mustered the courage to strike up a conversation with them. As they exchanged stories, she discovered that their contentment stemmed not from material possessions or fleeting successes, but from the simple yet profound changes they had made in their lives – changes that transformed their habits, their perspectives, and ultimately, their happiness. That encounter was a turning point for Sarah. It ignited a spark within her, a yearning to uncover the secrets of a truly happy life. She embarked on a journey of self-discovery, immersing herself in books, research, and personal experiences, all in pursuit of the path to a happier existence.

And now, dear reader, I invite you to join Sarah on this transformative journey. In "The Path to a Happier Life: Making Simple Changes for Healthy Habits," we will explore the profound connection between our habits and our happiness. We will delve into the power of small, intentional changes that have the potential to create a ripple effect in our lives, leading us toward a greater sense of fulfillment and joy.

The Importance of Happiness:

Happiness. It's a word that carries immense weight and yet often feels elusive, as if it were a distant island waiting to be discovered. We all desire it, yearn for it, and chase after it relentlessly. But why is happiness so important?

The truth is, happiness is not just a fleeting emotion or a momentary burst of joy. It is a state of being, a profound sense of well-being that permeates every aspect of our lives. When we are truly happy, we radiate positivity, compassion, and resilience. Our relationships flourish, our work becomes purposeful, and our overall health improves.

Numerous studies have shown the remarkable impact of happiness on our physical and mental well-being. It boosts our immune system, reduces stress levels, and enhances cognitive function. Happy individuals are more likely to lead fulfilling lives, achieve their goals, and experience greater overall satisfaction. Beyond its benefits, happiness has a ripple effect on the world around us. When we are genuinely content, we inspire others to pursue their happiness. We become beacons of light, spreading joy and kindness wherever we go. In a world that often feels overwhelmed by negativity, cultivating happiness becomes a powerful act of resilience and hope.

The Connection between Habits and Happiness:

Imagine our habits as the building blocks of our lives – the daily rituals, routines, and behaviors that shape who we are and what we experience. Now, consider this: if happiness is our ultimate destination, then our habits are the compass that guides us there.

Our habits influence not only our physical and mental well-being but also the lens through which we perceive the world. Positive habits, such as practicing gratitude, engaging in regular exercise, and nurturing meaningful relationships, can foster happiness and well-being. Conversely, negative habits, such as procrastination, self-doubt, and unhealthy coping mechanisms, can hinder our happiness.

By understanding the connection between habits and happiness, we can consciously create positive routines that bring us closer to a joyful and purposeful existence.

The Goal of the Book

The goal of this book is to empower you with the knowledge, tools, and practical strategies to make simple changes in your life that will lead to healthier habits and ultimately, a happier life. It is not about drastic transformations or overnight success, but rather about embracing a series of incremental changes that will have a lasting impact on your well-being.

Through the chapters that follow, we will explore various aspects of your life and provide guidance on how to nurture a positive mindset, prioritize physical health, enhance emotional well-being, create a supportive environment, embrace mindfulness and self-care, foster personal growth and learning, cultivate gratitude, and sustain healthy habits for the long term.

Each chapter will offer insights, actionable steps, and practical exercises to help you integrate healthy habits into your daily routine. It is important to remember that everyone's journey is unique, and what works for one person may not work for another. The key is to adapt and personalize the strategies to fit your lifestyle and preferences.

By embarking on this journey towards a happier life, you are taking a significant step towards self-care, self-improvement, and self-discovery. It won't always be easy, but the rewards will be immeasurable. Let's begin our journey together and unlock the secrets to a happier and more fulfilling life.

Daily Healthy Habits

Exercise > 9thousand steps

Quality sleep > 8hours of sleep

Hydration > 7glasses of water

Mediation > 6mins of mediation

Healthy eating > 5servings of fruit & veggies

Healthy eating > 3meals & 3healthy snacks

CHAPTER ONE

UNDERSTANDING HAPPINESS

By adopting strategies and habits that promote well-being, nurturing positive emotions, and prioritizing meaningful connections and activities, individuals can enhance their happiness and lead more fulfilling lives.

What is Happiness:

Happiness is a complex and subjective emotion that encompasses a state of well-being, contentment, and joy. It is a positive and pleasurable experience that brings a sense of fulfillment and satisfaction in life. While the concept of happiness can vary from person to person, it generally involves a combination of positive emotions, a sense of purpose or meaning, and overall life satisfaction. Happiness is not solely dependent on external circumstances but also influenced by internal factors such as mindset, values, and personal fulfillment.

The Science of Happiness:

The science of happiness, also known as positive psychology, is a field of study that focuses on understanding and promoting well-being and happiness. It utilizes scientific methods to explore the factors that contribute to happiness, the underlying mechanisms that influence our emotional states, and strategies for enhancing well-being.

Researchers in the field of positive psychology have identified several key components of happiness, such as positive emotions, engagement in meaningful activities, building and maintaining strong relationships, finding a sense of purpose and meaning in life, and also practicing gratitude and mindfulness. They have conducted studies and experiments to uncover the factors that contribute to long-term happiness, including genetics, personality traits, life circumstances, and intentional actions and habits.

The Benefits of Happiness:

Happiness is not only a desirable emotional state but also brings numerous benefits to various aspects of our lives. Research has consistently shown that cultivating happiness can have a positive impact on our overall well-being, physical health, mental health, relationships, and even success in various domains.

- **Physical Health:** Happiness is linked to better physical health outcomes. Happy individuals tend to have lower stress levels, stronger immune systems, lower blood pressure, reduced risk of cardiovascular disease, and faster recovery from illnesses.

- **Mental Health:** Happiness plays a crucial role in mental well-being. It is associated with lower rates of depression, anxiety, and other mental health disorders. Happy individuals tend to have higher resilience, better coping mechanisms, and improved emotional well-being.

- **Relationships:** Happiness is closely connected to fulfilling and satisfying relationships. Happy individuals are more likely to form and maintain strong social connections, experience deeper and more meaningful relationships, and have better communication and conflict-resolution skills.

- **Success and Productivity:** Happiness is not just a consequence of success but also a predictor of it. Research suggests that happy individuals are more motivated, creative, and productive. They tend to have better job satisfaction, higher income, and greater career success.

- **Overall Well-being and Quality of Life:** Happiness contributes to an overall sense of well-being and a higher quality of life. Happy individuals report greater life satisfaction, higher self-esteem, a greater sense of purpose and meaning, and a more positive outlook on life.

CHAPTER TWO

CHAPTER TWO

IDENTIFYING UNHEALTHY HABITS

Identifying unhealthy habits involves recognizing and becoming aware of patterns of behavior that have negative effects on your physical, mental, or emotional well-being. It is an essential step towards making positive changes and fostering a healthier lifestyle.

Common Unhealthy Habits:

Unhealthy habits are patterns of behavior that have negative effects on our physical, mental, or emotional well-being. They often involve actions that provide temporary gratification but can lead to long-term consequences. Some common unhealthy habits include:

- **Sedentary Lifestyle:** Engaging in a sedentary lifestyle, such as sitting for prolonged periods or lacking regular physical activity, can contribute to various health issues like obesity, heart disease, and weakened muscles and bones.

- **Poor Diet:** Consuming a diet high in processed foods, sugary snacks, unhealthy fats, and lacking essential nutrients can lead to weight gain, nutritional deficiencies, increased risk of chronic diseases, and low energy levels.

- **Excessive Consumption of Alcohol:** Regularly consuming excessive amounts of alcohol can result in liver damage, addiction, impaired judgment, relationship problems, and a range of physical and mental health issues.

- **Smoking:** Smoking tobacco products damages the lungs, and increases the risk of various cancers, heart disease, and respiratory problems. It also negatively impacts the health of those exposed to secondhand smoke.

- **Inadequate Sleep:** Consistently getting insufficient sleep can lead to fatigue, decreased cognitive function, a weakened immune system, mood swings, and an increased risk of accidents.

<u>The Consequences of Unhealthy Habits:</u>

Unhealthy habits can have significant consequences on our overall well-being. They can lead to:

- **Physical Health Issues:** Unhealthy habits contribute to a range of physical health problems, including obesity, cardiovascular diseases, diabetes, respiratory issues, weakened immune system, and increased risk of certain cancers.

- **Mental and Emotional Health Problems:** Unhealthy habits can negatively impact our mental and emotional well-being. They can contribute to increased stress levels, anxiety, depression, low self-esteem, decreased cognitive function, and impaired overall mental health.

- **Relationship Challenges:** Unhealthy habits can strain relationships with family, friends, and colleagues. They can lead to conflicts, lack of trust, and difficulties in maintaining healthy connections.

- **Decreased Quality of Life:** Unhealthy habits can diminish our overall quality of life. They can limit our energy levels, impair our ability to engage in activities we enjoy, reduce productivity, and hinder personal growth and fulfillment.

<u>*Identifying Personal Unhealthy Habits:*</u>

To identify your unhealthy habits, it is helpful to take a reflective and honest approach. Here are some steps to identify your unhealthy habits:

- **Self-Reflection:** Take time to reflect on your daily routines, behaviors, and choices. Consider areas where you feel dissatisfied or notice patterns that may be detrimental to your well-being.

- **Objective Evaluation:** Assess your habits objectively by considering the impact they have on your physical health, mental well-being, relationships, and overall functioning. Look for habits that consistently lead to negative consequences.

- **Seek Feedback:** Ask trusted friends, family members, or professionals for their observations and insights. They may provide valuable perspectives on habits that you may be unaware of or underestimate their impact.

- **Track and Monitor:** Keep a journal or use habit-tracking apps to record your behaviors and identify patterns. This can help you

become more aware of your habits and their
effects.

- **Emotional and Physical Indicators**: Pay
  attention to any emotional or physical signs
  that may indicate unhealthy habits. These
  could include feelings of guilt, fatigue, stress,
  changes in weight, or overall well-being.

Identifying unhealthy habits is an ongoing process
that requires self-awareness, honesty, and a
willingness to change. By recognizing and
acknowledging these habits, you can take proactive
steps towards replacing them with healthier
alternatives. Remember, self-compassion and
patience are essential during this process, as
breaking old habits and forming new ones takes time
and effort.

CHAPTER THREE

CREATING HEALTHY HABITS

Creating healthy habits involves intentionally adopting behaviors that promote your physical, mental, and emotional well-being. These habits are sustainable, positive routines that contribute to your overall health and happiness. They are actions and choices that align with your values and long-term goals.

The Importance of Healthy Habits:

Healthy habits play a crucial role in promoting overall well-being and leading a happier, more fulfilling life. Here are some key reasons why healthy habits are important:

- **Physical Health:** Healthy habits, such as regular exercise, a balanced diet, and sufficient sleep, contribute to better physical health. They help maintain a healthy weight, strengthen the immune system, reduce the risk of chronic diseases like heart disease and diabetes, and increase overall vitality.

- **Mental and Emotional Well-being**: Healthy habits positively impact mental and emotional health. Engaging in activities like mindfulness, practicing gratitude, and seeking social connections can enhance emotional resilience, reduce stress levels, improve mood, and promote a sense of overall well-being.

- **Energy and Productivity**: When we prioritize healthy habits, we increase our energy levels, mental clarity, and focus. This leads to improved productivity, better concentration, and the ability to effectively manage daily tasks and responsibilities.

- **Long-Term Well-being**: Healthy habits are sustainable practices that contribute to long-term well-being. By incorporating them into our daily routines, we create a foundation for a healthier and more fulfilling life, reducing the likelihood of experiencing health issues and improving our overall quality of life.

The Science of Habit Formation:

Habits are automatic behaviors that we perform without conscious effort or deliberation. The science of habit formation explores how habits are formed, maintained, and changed. Understanding the science behind habits can help us develop healthier habits effectively. Key principles of habit formation include:

-   **Cue-Routine-Reward:** Habits consist of a cue, a routine, and a reward. The cue triggers the behavior, the routine is the behavior itself, and the reward is the positive reinforcement that reinforces the habit loop.

-   **Habit Loop:** Habits are formed through repetition and reinforcement. When we consistently engage in a behavior and receive a reward, our brain forms neural connections that make the habit more automatic and ingrained.

-   **Habit Stacking:** Building on existing habits can make it easier to develop new ones. By associating a new habit with an existing one, we can leverage the existing habit as a cue and increase the likelihood of performing the new behavior.

-   **Environment and Context:** Our environment and the context in which we engage in behaviors significantly influence habit formation. Creating an environment that supports and encourages healthy habits can increase the chances of success.

<u>*Strategies for developing healthy habits:*</u>

- **Set Clear and Specific Goals:** Define the specific habits you want to develop and establish clear goals related to them. Make your goals realistic, measurable, and time-bound. For example, if you want to develop a habit of regular exercise, set a goal to exercise for 30 minutes, five times a week.

- **Start Small and Build Momentum:** Begin with small, achievable steps. Trying to change too much at once can be overwhelming and unsustainable. Focus on one habit at a time and gradually build upon your successes. As you experience small victories, it will boost your confidence and motivation to tackle more challenging habits.

- **Make it a Routine:** Consistency is key to establishing habits. Incorporate your desired behavior into your daily routine. Set specific times or cues that remind you to engage in the habit. Over time, it will become automatic and require less effort and willpower.

- **Create Accountability:** Find ways to hold yourself accountable for your habits. Share your goals and progress with supportive friends, family, or a mentor. Consider joining a group or finding an accountability partner who shares similar goals. Tracking your progress or using habit-tracking apps can also help maintain accountability.

- **Make it Enjoyable:** Find ways to make your healthy habits enjoyable. If you dread an activity, it will be challenging to sustain. Incorporate elements of fun, creativity, or variety into your habits. For example, if you want to eat healthier, explore new recipes, try different cuisines, or involve friends in meal planning and cooking.

- **Overcome Obstacles:** Identify potential obstacles that may hinder your habit development and plan strategies to overcome them. Anticipate challenges and have contingency plans in place. For instance, if you have a busy schedule, identify shorter workout routines or find ways to incorporate physical activity into your daily routine, such as taking the stairs instead of the elevator.

- **Practice Mindfulness and Self-Reflection:** Cultivate awareness of your thoughts, emotions, and behaviors. Regularly reflect on your progress, challenges, and successes. Celebrate your achievements and learn from setbacks. Mindfulness can help you stay present, make conscious choices, and stay committed to your healthy habits.

- **Seek Support and Resources:** Utilize available resources to support your habit development. Read books, and articles, or attend workshops related to your desired habits. Seek guidance from professionals, such as trainers, coaches, or therapists. Engage in online communities or forums that focus on healthy habits for support and inspiration.

Remember, developing healthy habits takes time and effort. Be patient with yourself and embrace the journey. Focus on progress rather than perfection. With consistent practice and a positive mindset, you can gradually replace unhealthy habits with sustainable and life-enhancing behaviors.

CHAPTER FOUR

PHYSICAL HEALTH HABITS

Physical health habits encompass actions and routines that contribute to the maintenance and enhancement of physical well-being. These habits play a role in optimizing physical functioning, preventing illness and disease, and supporting overall vitality.

Exercise:

Exercise involves engaging in physical activity to improve or sustain physical fitness and overall health. It entails planned, structured, and repetitive movements that target different areas of the body. Regular exercise provides numerous benefits for both physical and mental well-being. Here are key aspects of exercise:

Physical Benefits:

- **Enhanced cardiovascular health**: Exercise strengthens the heart, improves blood circulation, and reduces the risk of cardiovascular diseases.

- **Weight management:** Regular exercise helps in maintaining a healthy weight by burning calories and increasing metabolism.

- **Strengthened muscles and bones:** Exercise promotes muscle strength, endurance, and bone density, reducing the risk of osteoporosis and enhancing overall physical strength.

- **Increased flexibility and mobility:** Specific exercises such as stretching or yoga improve flexibility, joint range of motion, and balance.

- **Heightened energy levels:** Exercise boosts energy levels by enhancing the delivery of oxygen and nutrients to tissues, improving stamina, and reducing fatigue.

- **Improved immune system:** Regular exercise has been proven to enhance immune function and lower the risk of certain illnesses.

Mental and Emotional Benefits:

- **Reduced stress and anxiety:** Exercise helps release endorphins, natural mood-boosting chemicals that lead to reduced stress and anxiety.

- **Enhanced mental health:** Regular physical activity can alleviate symptoms of depression, improve self-esteem, enhance cognitive function, and promote better sleep.

- **Increased relaxation and better sleep:** Engaging in exercise promotes relaxation, reduces insomnia, and improves sleep quality.

Nutrition:

Nutrition refers to the process of acquiring and consuming food that provides the body with essential nutrients required for optimal functioning and well-being. A balanced and nutritious diet plays a vital role in maintaining good health. Here are key aspects of nutrition:

Macronutrients:

- **Carbohydrates:** Primary source of energy for the body, found in foods such as grains, fruits, vegetables, and legumes.

- **Proteins:** Essential for growth, repair, and maintenance of body tissues, found in foods such as meat, poultry, fish, dairy, legumes, and nuts.

- **Fats:** Important for energy, insulation, and hormone production, found in foods such as oils, nuts, seeds, avocados, and fatty fish.

Micronutrients:

- **Vitamins**: Essential for various bodily functions, including metabolism, immune function, and cell production. Found in fruits, vegetables, whole grains, and dairy products.

- **Minerals:** Play a crucial role in maintaining fluid balance, forming bones, and facilitating enzymatic reactions. Found in foods such as leafy greens, nuts, seeds, and lean meats.

Importance of a Balanced Diet:

A balanced diet should include a variety of nutrient-dense foods from all food groups to ensure an adequate intake of essential nutrients.
It is crucial to consume appropriate portions and practice moderation in the consumption of foods high in added sugars, unhealthy fats, and sodium.

Hydration is also important, so it is recommended to drink an adequate amount of water throughout the day.

Sleep:

Sleep is a vital physiological process that plays an essential role in maintaining overall health and well-being. It is a natural state of rest during which the body undergoes important restorative processes. Here is everything you need to know about sleep:

- Sleep Stages:

Sleep consists of different stages that cycle throughout the night. These stages include non-rapid eye movement (NREM) sleep and rapid eye movement (REM) sleep. NREM sleep is further divided into three stages, with each stage representing a different depth of sleep.

- Sleep Duration:

The recommended amount of sleep varies depending on age and individual needs. Adults generally require between 7 to 9 hours of sleep per night, while infants and children need more sleep for proper growth and development.

- <u>**Importance of Sleep:**</u>

Sleep is crucial for various aspects of physical and mental health. It plays a vital role in memory consolidation, learning, cognitive function, mood regulation, immune system function, hormone regulation, and overall cellular repair and rejuvenation.

- <u>**Consequences of Sleep Deprivation:**</u>

Lack of sufficient sleep can have significant consequences on physical and mental well-being. Sleep deprivation is associated with decreased cognitive function, impaired memory, reduced concentration, increased risk of accidents, weakened immune system, mood disturbances, and increased risk of chronic conditions like obesity, diabetes, and cardiovascular disease.

- <u>**Sleep Hygiene:**</u>

Good sleep hygiene refers to healthy habits and practices that promote quality sleep. This includes maintaining a consistent sleep schedule, creating a comfortable sleep environment (cool, dark, and quiet), limiting exposure to electronic devices before bed, avoiding stimulants like caffeine close to bedtime, and engaging in relaxing activities before sleep.

- ### *Common Sleep Disorders:*

Several sleep disorders can disrupt sleep patterns and quality. Some common sleep disorders include insomnia (difficulty falling asleep or staying asleep), sleep apnea (breathing interruptions during sleep), restless legs syndrome (uncomfortable sensations in the legs), and narcolepsy (excessive daytime sleepiness).

CHAPTER FIVE

EMOTIONAL HEALTH HABITS

Emotional health habits refer to the practices and behaviors that promote and maintain emotional well-being. These habits can help individuals develop resilience, cope with stress, and enhance their overall emotional health. Here are some key emotional health habits:

- **Self-awareness:** Being aware of your emotions, thoughts, and reactions is essential for emotional well-being. Take time to reflect on your feelings, identify triggers, and understand how they impact your mental state.

- **Stress management:** Effective stress management techniques are crucial for emotional health. Engage in activities that help you relax and unwind, such as exercise, deep breathing, meditation, or engaging in hobbies you enjoy.

- **Healthy coping mechanisms:** Rather than resorting to unhealthy coping mechanisms like substance abuse or avoidance, develop healthy ways to deal with difficult emotions. This could include talking to a supportive friend or family member, seeking therapy or counseling, or expressing yourself through creative outlets like writing or art.

- **Social connections:** Building and nurturing positive relationships is vital for emotional health. Surround yourself with supportive people who uplift you, and make an effort to maintain healthy social connections. Engage in activities that foster social interaction and create a sense of belonging.

- **Self-care:** Prioritizing self-care is essential for emotional well-being. This involves taking care of your physical, mental, and emotional needs. Make time for activities you enjoy, get enough sleep, eat nutritious meals, and set boundaries to protect your overall well-being.

Self-Care:

Self-care is the intentional practice of taking care of oneself physically, mentally, and emotionally. It involves nurturing your well-being and engaging in activities that promote self-nourishment and rejuvenation. Here are some key aspects of self-care:

-   **Physical self-care:** Engaging in activities that support your physical health, such as exercising regularly, eating nutritious foods, getting enough sleep, and attending to your personal hygiene needs.

-   **Emotional self-care:** Focusing on activities that enhance your emotional well-being, such as engaging in hobbies you enjoy, spending time with loved ones, seeking therapy or counseling when needed, and expressing your emotions in healthy ways.

-   **Mental self-care:** Take care of your mental health by engaging in activities that stimulate your mind, such as reading, learning new skills, practicing relaxation techniques, or engaging in creative outlets.

-   **Setting boundaries:** Establishing boundaries is a crucial aspect of self-care. Learn to say no to activities or commitments that overwhelm you and prioritize your own needs. Setting healthy boundaries helps prevent burnout and fosters a healthy work-life balance.

<u>*Mindfulness:*</u>

Mindfulness is the practice of intentionally bringing one's attention to the present moment without judgment. It involves being fully aware of your thoughts, emotions, bodily sensations, and the surrounding environment. Key aspects of mindfulness include:

* **Present-moment awareness:** Mindfulness emphasizes focusing on the here and now, rather than dwelling on the past or worrying about the future.

* **Non-judgmental attitude:** It involves observing your experiences without labeling them as good or bad, right or wrong.

* **Acceptance:** Mindfulness encourages accepting things as they are, including your thoughts and emotions, without trying to change or resist them.

* **Cultivating a beginner's mind:** This means approaching each experience with a sense of curiosity and openness as if it were the first time you were encountering it.

Mindfulness practices can include meditation, body scans, mindful eating, mindful walking, and mindful breathing exercises. Regular mindfulness practice has been shown to reduce stress, improve focus and attention, increase emotional regulation, and promote overall well-being.

Gratitude:

Gratitude is the practice of intentionally recognizing and appreciating the good things in one's life. It involves cultivating a positive outlook and acknowledging the blessings, big or small, that we often take for granted. Key aspects of gratitude include:

* **Recognition of abundance**: Gratitude helps shift our focus from what is lacking to what is already present in our lives.

* **Appreciation of the present moment**: It encourages noticing and savoring the positive experiences that are happening right now.

* **Cultivating positive emotions**: Expressing gratitude fosters feelings of joy, contentment, and happiness.

* **Connection and empathy**: Gratitude can enhance our relationships by fostering a sense of connection, empathy, and goodwill toward others.

Gratitude practices can include keeping a gratitude journal, writing thank-you notes, expressing appreciation to others, and reflecting on the positive aspects of each day. Research suggests that regular gratitude practice can improve mental health, enhance relationships, increase resilience, and promote a more positive outlook on life.

CHAPTER SIX

SOCIAL HEALTH HABITS

Social health habits are behaviors and practices that contribute to the development and maintenance of positive social relationships and overall social well-being. These habits involve engaging in healthy and fulfilling interactions with others, building and nurturing supportive networks and fostering a sense of belonging and connection. Here are some key social health habits:

-   **Communication**: Effective communication is essential for social health. It involves actively listening, expressing thoughts and feelings clearly, and being respectful of others' opinions. Good communication skills help establish and maintain healthy relationships.

-   **Active listening:** Actively listening to others means giving them your full attention, being present in the conversation, and showing genuine interest in what they have to say. It fosters understanding, empathy, and deeper connections with others.

- **Building and maintaining relationships:** Cultivating and nurturing relationships is important for social health. This involves investing time and effort into building connections, creating shared experiences, and offering support to others. It includes both personal relationships with family and friends and professional relationships with colleagues and acquaintances.

- **Boundaries:** Setting healthy boundaries in relationships is crucial. It involves defining what is acceptable and respectful in terms of personal space, time, and emotional well-being. Establishing boundaries helps maintain balance and prevent feelings of being overwhelmed or taken advantage of.

- **Empathy and compassion:** Developing empathy and compassion involves understanding and sharing the feelings of others. It means being able to put yourself in someone else's shoes and respond with kindness, support, and understanding. These qualities enhance social connections and contribute to a positive social environment.

- **Conflict resolution:** Conflict is a natural part of relationships, but resolving conflicts in a healthy and constructive manner is vital for social health. Effective conflict resolution involves active listening, expressing concerns calmly, finding mutually agreeable solutions, and being open to compromise.

- **Active participation in the community:** Engaging in community activities and being an active participant in social groups can greatly enhance social health. It provides opportunities to connect with others, contribute to the community, and foster a sense of belonging and purpose.

- **Support networks:** Building and maintaining a supportive network of friends, family, and colleagues is essential for social health. These networks provide emotional support, companionship, and a sense of belonging, especially during challenging times.

- **Positive social media use:** Social media can play a role in social health when used in a positive and mindful way. It can help connect with others, share experiences, and maintain relationships. However, it's important to balance online interactions with real-life connections and be mindful of the impact of social media on mental well-being.

By incorporating these social health habits into daily life, individuals can foster positive social connections, strengthen relationships, and enhance overall well-being. Good social health contributes to a sense of belonging, support, and happiness, and it is an important aspect of leading a fulfilling and meaningful life.

Building Strong Relationships:

Building strong relationships is essential for personal and social well-being. Building strong relationships provide support, companionship, and a sense of belonging. Here are some key elements of building strong relationships:

- **Trust:** Trust forms the foundation of any strong relationship. It involves being reliable, and honest, and maintaining confidentiality. Trust is built over time through consistent actions and open communication.

- **Effective communication:** Communication is crucial for building strong relationships. It involves active listening, expressing thoughts and feelings clearly, and being respectful of others' perspectives. Good communication helps foster understanding, resolve conflicts, and build a deeper connection.

- **Emotional support:** Strong relationships involve providing emotional support to one another. This includes offering empathy, understanding, and validation when someone is going through difficult times. Being there for each other and offering a shoulder to lean on strengthens the bond.

- **Shared values and interests:** Common values and interests help create a sense of shared purpose and connection. Engaging in activities or hobbies together fosters shared experiences and strengthens the bond between individuals.

- **Quality time:** Spending quality time together is vital for building strong relationships. This includes engaging in meaningful conversations, creating memories, and enjoying each other's company. Making time for one another demonstrates care and commitment.

<u>*Communication Skills:*</u>

Effective communication skills are essential for establishing and maintaining healthy relationships. Here are some key communication skills:

- **Active listening:** Active listening involves fully focusing on and understanding what the other person is saying. It includes maintaining eye contact, nodding or providing verbal cues to show engagement, and avoiding interrupting or judgment.

- **Clarity and assertiveness:** Clearly expressing thoughts, feelings, and needs help prevent misunderstandings and promotes effective communication. Being assertive involves respectfully expressing oneself while considering the feelings and perspectives of others.

- **Non-verbal communication:** Non-verbal cues, such as body language, facial expressions, and tone of voice, play a significant role in communication. Being aware of and using appropriate non-verbal cues enhances understanding and connection.

- **Empathy**: Empathy involves understanding and sharing the emotions and experiences of others. It helps foster a deeper connection and demonstrates that you value and care about the other person's feelings.

- **Conflict resolution**: Conflict is a normal part of relationships, and having the skills to resolve conflicts constructively is crucial. This includes active listening, expressing concerns calmly, finding compromises, and seeking win-win solutions.

<u>*Cultivating Positive Social Interactions:*</u>

Positive social interactions contribute to a sense of happiness, well-being, and social connectedness. Here are some ways to cultivate positive social interactions:

1. **Kindness and respect:** Treating others with kindness, respect, and consideration creates a positive social environment. Small acts of kindness and politeness can go a long way in fostering positive interactions.

2. **Active participation:** Actively participate in social activities, groups, or community events that align with your interests. This allows for

opportunities to meet new people, engage in shared experiences, and foster positive connections.

3. **Genuine interest:** Show genuine interest in others by asking questions, actively listening, and engaging in conversations. This demonstrates that you value their perspectives and helps create a positive and meaningful interaction.

4. **Positive attitude:** Cultivate a positive attitude and outlook when interacting with others. Positivity is contagious and can contribute to a positive and uplifting social atmosphere.

5. **Empathy and compassion:** Practice empathy and compassion toward others. This involves understanding and acknowledging their emotions, offering support, and showing understanding and kindness.

By incorporating these principles into your relationships and social interactions, you can build strong connections, enhance communication skills, and cultivate positive and fulfilling social experiences.

CHAPTER SEVEN

MAINTAINING HEALTHY HABITS

Maintaining healthy habits is consistently practicing behaviors and routines that promote physical, mental, and emotional well-being. It involves making conscious choices and taking proactive steps to sustain healthy habits over time. Here are some key aspects of maintaining healthy habits:

- **Consistency:** Consistency is vital for maintaining healthy habits. It involves making a commitment to engage in healthy behaviors regularly and sticking to them even when faced with challenges or setbacks. Consistency helps solidify habits and ensures long-term benefits.

- **Goal setting:** Setting specific, realistic, and achievable goals is crucial for maintaining healthy habits. Goals provide motivation and a sense of purpose. Break down large goals into smaller, manageable steps to make progress and stay motivated.

- **Self-discipline:** Self-discipline plays a significant role in maintaining healthy habits.

It involves making conscious choices and resisting temptations that may hinder progress. Developing self-discipline requires practice and cultivating a mindset of self-control and determination.

- **Accountability:** Holding yourself accountable or seeking external accountability can help maintain healthy habits. This can be done by tracking progress, sharing goals with a trusted friend or family member, or joining a supportive community or group that shares similar health goals.

- **Flexibility and adaptation:** Maintaining healthy habits also requires flexibility and the ability to adapt to changing circumstances. Life is dynamic, and being able to adjust your habits when needed ensures their sustainability. Modify your routines and strategies to accommodate new situations without compromising the overall goal.

- **Self-care and stress management:** Prioritizing self-care and managing stress are essential for maintaining healthy habits. Make time for activities that recharge and rejuvenate you, such as exercise, relaxation techniques,

hobbies, and quality sleep. Managing stress
helps prevent burnout and supports overall
well-being.

- **Positive mindset and self-compassion:**
Cultivate a positive mindset and practice self-
compassion when maintaining healthy habits.
Embrace a growth mindset, and prioritize
focusing on progress rather than perfection.
Treat yourself with kindness and
understanding, celebrating achievements and
learning from setbacks.

- **Support system:** Building a support system
can greatly aid in maintaining healthy habits.
Surround yourself with individuals who
encourage and support your goals. Seek out
friends, family, or communities that share
similar interests or health goals, as they can
provide motivation, accountability, and a
sense of belonging.

- **Reflect and reassess:** Regularly reflect on your
habits and assess their effectiveness. Take
time to evaluate your progress, identify areas
for improvement, and make necessary
adjustments. Reflecting and reassessing your

habits ensure that they remain aligned with your current needs and goals.

Remember that maintaining healthy habits is an ongoing process that requires commitment, effort, and a positive mindset. By incorporating these principles into your daily life and staying consistent, you can cultivate a sustainable and fulfilling lifestyle that supports your overall well-being.

Overcoming Obstacles:

Overcoming obstacles refers to the ability to navigate challenges, setbacks, and difficulties in order to achieve desired goals. It involves developing resilience, problem-solving skills, and a positive mindset. Here are some key aspects of overcoming obstacles:

- **Resilience:** Resilience is the ability to bounce back from setbacks and adapt to change. It includes developing a mindset that views obstacles as opportunities for growth and learning rather than barriers. Building resilience requires developing coping mechanisms, seeking support, and maintaining a positive outlook.

- **Problem-solving skills:** Developing effective problem-solving skills is essential for overcoming obstacles. It involves identifying the problem, exploring potential solutions, and taking action to address the issue. Being proactive, resourceful, and open to new approaches can help overcome obstacles more effectively.

- **Persistence and determination:** Overcoming obstacles often requires persistence and determination. It involves staying committed to the goal, even in the face of challenges or setbacks. Having a strong sense of purpose and motivation can help maintain the drive to overcome obstacles.

- **Flexibility and adaptability:** Being flexible and adaptable is important when faced with obstacles. It involves adjusting strategies and approaches as needed to overcome challenges. Embracing change and being open to alternative solutions can increase the likelihood of success.

- **Learning from setbacks:** Viewing setbacks as learning opportunities is crucial for overcoming obstacles. Instead of getting discouraged, reflect on the experience, identify lessons learned, and apply them to future endeavors. This allows for personal growth and improvement.

The Power of Accountability:

The power of accountability lies in taking responsibility for one's actions, commitments, and goals. Being accountable involves being answerable to oneself and others, which can significantly impact personal growth and goal achievement. Here's why accountability is powerful:

1. **Motivation and focus:** Being accountable to yourself or others provides motivation and focus. Knowing that you have commitments and someone to report to can increase your determination and drive to follow through on your goals.

2. **Commitment and consistency:** Accountability helps promote commitment and consistency in pursuing your goals. When you're accountable, you're more likely to stay on track and follow through on your plans and actions.

3. **Support and feedback:** Accountability often involves involving others who can provide support, guidance, and feedback. This support system can offer encouragement, share knowledge and resources, and provide constructive criticism to help you stay on the right path.

4. **Identifying obstacles and finding solutions:** Being accountable requires recognizing obstacles or challenges that may hinder progress. This awareness allows you to take proactive steps to overcome obstacles, seek assistance when needed, and find solutions to stay on track.

5. **Celebration of achievements:** Accountability also helps celebrate achievements along the way. Sharing progress and accomplishments with others who hold you accountable reinforces positive behavior and provides a sense of accomplishment and satisfaction.

<u>Self-compassion:</u>

Self-compassion involves treating oneself with kindness, care, and understanding, especially in moments of difficulty, failure, or suffering. It involves extending the same compassion and empathy towards oneself that one would offer to a loved one or a close friend. Self-compassion encompasses three key components:

1. **Self-kindness**: Self-kindness involves being gentle and understanding towards oneself rather than self-critical or judgmental. It means responding to personal failures or shortcomings with empathy, patience, and a nurturing attitude.

2. **Common humanity:** Recognizing the shared human experience of suffering and imperfection is an essential aspect of self-compassion. It involves understanding that everyone faces challenges, makes mistakes, and experiences pain, rather than feeling isolated or inadequate.

3. **Mindfulness:** Mindfulness is the practice of being aware of the present moment without judgment. In the context of self-compassion, mindfulness involves acknowledging and accepting one's emotions, thoughts, and experiences without suppressing or exaggerating them.

<u>**_The Role of Self-compassion in personal well-being:_**</u>

- **Emotional well-being:** Self-compassion promotes emotional well-being by fostering self-acceptance, self-love, and self-worth. It allows individuals to embrace their strengths and weaknesses without harsh self-criticism, leading to greater emotional resilience, reduced stress, and improved overall mental health.

- **Reduced self-criticism and perfectionism:** Self-compassion helps counteract self-critical and perfectionistic tendencies. It allows individuals to embrace their imperfections and failures as part of the human experience, reducing the pressure to constantly achieve and meet unrealistic standards.

- **Resilience and coping with adversity:** Self-compassion supports resilience by providing individuals with a compassionate mindset when facing adversity or setbacks. It helps individuals bounce back from failures, learn from mistakes, and navigate challenging situations with self-care and understanding.

- **Improved relationships:** Practicing self-compassion can positively impact relationships with others. When individuals are kinder to themselves, they tend to be more understanding, empathetic, and compassionate towards others. It promotes healthier and more fulfilling social connections.

- **Motivation and personal growth:** Contrary to self-criticism, self-compassion fuels motivation and personal growth. By embracing themselves with kindness and understanding, individuals feel safer taking risks, exploring new opportunities, and learning from experiences without fear of harsh self-judgment.

- **Physical well-being:** Self-compassion has been linked to improved physical health outcomes. It reduces the detrimental effects of chronic stress, supports healthier lifestyle choices, and promotes self-care behaviors such as exercise, balanced nutrition, and sufficient sleep.

Overall, self-compassion plays a vital role in personal well-being by cultivating a kinder and more nurturing relationship with oneself. It enhances emotional resilience, fosters healthy self-esteem, and contributes to a more balanced and fulfilling life.

Developing and maintaining healthy habits is a powerful way to enhance various aspects of life. By prioritizing physical, mental, and emotional well-being, individuals can experience a range of benefits and pave the path to a happier life. Building strong relationships, honing communication skills, cultivating positive social interactions, and overcoming obstacles are essential components of personal growth and fulfillment. Embracing the power of accountability and self-compassion further supports overall well-being and resilience. With dedication, consistency, and a positive mindset, anyone can embark on a transformative journey toward a healthier, happier, and more fulfilling life.

The Benefits of Healthy Habits:

Adopting and maintaining healthy habits brings numerous benefits that positively impact every aspect of life. Some key benefits include:

- **Physical well-being:** Healthy habits such as regular exercise, balanced nutrition, and sufficient sleep contribute to improved physical health, higher energy levels, and a reduced risk of chronic diseases.

- **Mental and emotional well-being:** Engaging in self-care practices, managing stress, and nurturing positive relationships enhance mental and emotional well-being. Healthy habits can lead to reduced anxiety and depression, improved mood, increased self-confidence, and better overall psychological health.

- **Productivity and focus:** When the body and mind are nourished through healthy habits, individuals experience increased productivity, improved concentration, and enhanced cognitive function. This enables better performance in various areas of life, including work, studies, and personal pursuits.

- **Longevity and quality of life:** By adopting healthy habits, individuals increase their chances of living longer and healthier life. Healthy behaviors such as regular exercise, a nutritious diet, and stress management contribute to overall longevity and a higher quality of life as individuals age.

<u>**The Path to a Happier Life:**</u>

A happier life is attainable by incorporating certain practices and perspectives into one's daily routine. Here are some elements that contribute to a happier life:

- **Gratitude:** Cultivating gratitude and appreciating the positive aspects of life can lead to increased happiness and contentment. Taking time to acknowledge and express gratitude for the blessings, experiences, and relationships fosters a positive outlook.

- **Mindfulness:** Practicing mindfulness involves being fully present in the current moment, without judgment or attachment. It helps individuals develop a deeper sense of awareness, reduce stress, and find joy in simple pleasures.

- **Pursuing passions:** Engaging in activities and hobbies that bring joy and fulfillment adds meaning to life. By pursuing passions, individuals tap into their unique talents and interests, fostering a sense of purpose and satisfaction.

- **Meaningful relationships:** Nurturing meaningful relationships and social connections is crucial for happiness. Building strong relationships, fostering open communication, and investing time in nurturing connections with loved ones contribute to a happier and more fulfilling life.

- **Self-care:** Prioritizing self-care and well-being is essential for a happier life. Taking care of physical, mental, and emotional needs, setting boundaries, and engaging in activities that recharge and rejuvenate promotes a sense of balance and happiness.

Final Thoughts and Encouragement:

Embarking on a journey toward a healthier and happier life requires commitment, effort, and self-compassion. Remember that change takes time and setbacks are part of the process. Embrace the power of resilience, accountability, and self-compassion to navigate obstacles and stay on track. Celebrate every small victory along the way and acknowledge the progress made. Surround yourself with supportive people who uplift and encourage you. Take small steps, set realistic goals, and make choices that align with your values and aspirations. With perseverance and a positive mindset, you can create a life filled with joy, fulfillment, and well-being. Believe in your potential and trust the process as you embark on this transformative journey.

GROWTH CHALLENGE TO CONSIDER TO BE ON THE PATH OF A HAPPIER LIFE

Making your well-being a priority is not selfish; it's necessary. Take time to nourish your body, mind, and soul. Make self-care activities like exercising, eating nutritious meals, getting enough sleep, and engaging in hobbies a regular part of your routine.

The 60-day challenge for "The Path to a Happier Life":

Week 1: Self-Reflection and Mindfulness

- Day 1: Start a gratitude journal. Write down three things you're grateful for each day.
- Day 2: Practice deep breathing exercises for 10 minutes to reduce stress.
- Day 3: Spend 15 minutes in meditation or mindfulness practice.
- Day 4: Write down your goals and aspirations for a happier life.
- Day 5: Take a break from social media and engage in a hobby you enjoy.
- Day 6: Practice positive affirmations and repeat them throughout the day.

- Day 7: Reflect on your progress during the first week and identify areas for improvement.

<u>Week 2: Physical Health and Fitness</u>

- Day 8: Start your day with a healthy breakfast, including fruits and whole grains.
- Day 9: Go for a 30-minute walk or engage in any physical activity you enjoy.
- Day 10: Drink at least 8 glasses of water throughout the day.
- Day 11: Try a new healthy recipe for lunch or dinner.
- Day 12: Replace sugary snacks with nutritious alternatives like fruits or nuts.
- Day 13: Incorporate stretching exercises into your daily routine.
- Day 14: Reflect on your physical health and set achievable fitness goals.

<u>Week 3: Emotional Well-being</u>

- Day 15: Write a letter to yourself, acknowledging your strengths and achievements.
- Day 16: Practice forgiveness—let go of grudges or negative feelings towards others.

-   Day 17: Reach out to a friend or loved one and
    express your appreciation.
-   Day 18: Engage in a creative activity that
    brings you joy, like painting or writing.
-   Day 19: Watch or read something inspirational
    that uplifts your mood.
-   Day 20: Practice acts of kindness, such as
    helping someone in need.
-   Day 21: Reflect on your emotional well-being
    and find ways to cultivate positivity.

Week 4: Social Connections

-   Day 22: Plan a social outing or gather with
    friends/family for a meaningful activity.
-   Day 23: Volunteer for a cause that resonates
    with you.
-   Day 24: Connect with a friend you haven't
    spoken to in a while.
-   Day 25: Practice active listening in
    conversations and show genuine interest.
-   Day 26: Attend a social event or join a
    club/organization to meet new people.
-   Day 27: Arrange a virtual hangout with friends
    or family members.
-   Day 28: Reflect on the value of your social
    connections and nurture them.

Week 5: Productivity and Time Management

- Day 29: Prioritize your tasks for the day and create a to-do list.
- Day 30: Eliminate distractions and allocate focused time for important tasks.
- Day 31: Practice the Pomodoro Technique—work in 25-minute intervals with breaks.
- Day 32: Delegate tasks that can be done by others to lighten your workload.
- Day 33: Organize your workspace or living area to enhance productivity.
- Day 34: Learn a new skill or take a course to expand your knowledge.
- Day 35: Reflect on your productivity habits and make adjustments if necessary.

Week 6: Mindful Consumption and Self-Care

- Day 36: Practice digital detox for a few hours and engage in offline activities.
- Day 37: Read a book or listen to a podcast that inspires personal growth and positivity.
- Day 38: Declutter your living space and create a more organized environment.

- Day 39: Try a new healthy recipe or explore a new cuisine for a nourishing meal.
- Day 40: Pamper yourself with a relaxing bath or indulge in a self-care activity of your choice.
- Day 41: Practice mindful eating by savoring each bite and paying attention to your body's hunger and fullness cues.
- Day 42: Engage in a hobby or activity that brings you joy and allows for creative expression.

Week 7: Gratitude and Kindness

- Day 43: Write a heartfelt thank-you note to someone who has positively impacted your life.
- Day 44: Practice random acts of kindness throughout the day, such as offering compliments or helping others.
- Day 45: Reflect on three things you appreciate about yourself and acknowledge your strengths.
- Day 46: Volunteer your time or skills to a charitable organization in your community.
- Day 47: Spend time in nature, appreciating the beauty and serenity it offers.

- Day 48: Express gratitude for the simple things in life, such as a warm cup of tea or a beautiful sunset.
- Day 49: Reflect on the power of gratitude and kindness in cultivating happiness and contentment.

Week 8: Reflection and Future Growth

- Day 50: Take time to reflect on the progress you have made throughout the 60-day challenge.
- Day 51: Set new goals for your continued personal growth and happiness journey.
- Day 52: Identify any areas for improvement or habits you would like to change moving forward.
- Day 53: Write a letter to your future self, outlining your aspirations and dreams.
- Day 54: Practice self-reflection through journaling, and exploring your thoughts, and emotions.
- Day 55-58: Reach out to a mentor or seek guidance to support your personal and professional development.
- 58. Day 58-60 Celebrate the completion of the 60-day challenge and acknowledge your commitment to a happier life.

Keep in mind that a healthy lifestyle is an investment in your future. Regular exercise, nutritious eating, and self-care habits contribute to your overall well-being, reduce the risk of chronic diseases, and increase your longevity. You're making positive choices that will pay off in the long run.

www.ingramcontent.com/pod-product-compliance
Lightning Source LLC
Chambersburg PA
CBHW051839250726
48659CB00005B/1921